Gastric Sleeve Cookbook

Delicious Recipes to Recover Yourself After Bariatric Weight Loss Surgery

Table of Contents

Introduction

Congratulations on downloading the *Gastric Sleeve Cookbook: Delicious Recipes to Recover Yourself After Bariatric Weight Loss Surgery*. Thank you for doing so.

You are making all of the right moves to improve your lifestyle. You will surely want to add *Gastric Sleeve Cookbook: Delicious Recipes to Recover Yourself After Bariatric Weight Loss Surgery* to your personal library. It will provide you with many new dishes you never thought would be possible to prepare and remain healthy.

You will soon discover within the pages of this cookbook that you are truly entering a new stage of your life. You have the tools to continue down the right path to a much healthier future.

These are just a few of the recipes you can enjoy:

- Chicken Creole
- Ranch Cheddar Turkey Burgers
- Mediterranean Salmon with Pasta
- Crunchy Tuna Patties
- Curried Carrot Soup
- Meatloaf Muffins
- Caramel Apple Salad
- Coconut Meringue Cookies

Plus, so much more!

The following chapters will discuss many ways to cook food you have always eaten. You will discover how many different ways you can cook beef, poultry, seafood, and many other foods. For most of the recipes it is important to use non-fat, reduced-sodium, and similar choices when they are available, since that is how you can easily reduce the calorie and carbohydrate intakes.

There are plenty of books on this subject on the market, thanks again for choosing this one! Every effort was made to ensure it is full of as much useful information as possible. Please enjoy!

Happy Cooking!

Chapter 1: Poultry and Turkey

Almond Chicken Salad with Asparagus

Ingredients
12 ounces cooked chicken breast- boneless and skinless
2 cups asparagus tips
1 teaspoon each:
- Fresh lemon juice
- Curry powder

½ cup plain, yogurt
1/8 teaspoon pepper
¼ teaspoon salt
¼ cup freshly chopped cilantro
½ cup red bell pepper (seeded and chopped)
Spinach leaves
2 tablespoons toasted sliced almonds

Instructions
1. Diagonally cut the asparagus and chop the chicken.
2. Steam the asparagus for two minutes.
3. Mix the lemon juice, salt, curry, pepper, and yogurt. Blend in the chicken asparagus, almonds, and cilantro. Toss to cover evenly and serve over the leaves of spinach.

Yields: Four servings
Cal: 161.5 | P: 24 g | C: 7.9 g | F: 4.1 g

Baked Chicken and Vegetables

Ingredients
6 sliced carrots
4 sliced potatoes
1 large quartered onion
1 skinless raw chicken

1 teaspoon thyme
½ cup water
¼ teaspoon pepper

Instructions
1. Set the oven temperature in advance to 400°F.
2. Arrange the carrots, potatoes, and onions in a roasting pan.
   Add the chicken last.
3. Combine the pepper, thyme, and water. Dump them over the ingredients in the pan.
4. Bake for one hour until brown and tender. Baste the chicken with the juices several times.

Yields: Six servings
Cal: 240 | P: 26 g | C: 25 g | F: 3.5g

Brown Sugar Garlic Chicken

Ingredients
12 ounces chicken breasts (no skins or bones)
1 garlic clove
2 tablespoons butter
Dash of black pepper
4 teaspoons brown sugar

Instructions
1. Melt the butter and add the garlic in a frying pan.
2. Add the chicken flavored with the pepper, and cook until done (about 15 minutes).
3. Sprinkle with the brown sugar, cook for five minutes, and serve.

Yields: Four servings
Cal: 166.4 | P: 19.4 g | C: 4.3 g | F: 8.0 g

Chicken and Broccoli Casserole

Ingredients
1 package broccoli spears (frozen - 10 ounces)
1 pound breast of chicken
1 can of (low sodium) cream of mushroom soup
3 tbsp. mayonnaise
1 cup shredded cheddar cheese

Instructions
1. Remove all bones and skin from the chicken. Boil and drain the chicken breasts. When cooled, cut into one-inch bits.
2. Add the soup and mayonnaise in a casserole dish. Blend in the chicken and broccoli, mixing well.
3. Dust with the cheese and bake for approximately twenty minutes.

Yields: Four servings
Cal: 284.2 | P: 36.8 g | C: 15.8 g | F: 7.3 g

Chicken Broccoli and Tomato Stir Fry

Ingredients
1 pound chicken breast (boneless - chopped
1 tbsp. soy sauce
2 tsp. canola oil
1 tsp. fresh ginger
¼ tsp. salt
2 tsp. finely chopped garlic
3 cups broccoli florets
4 firm plum tomatoes
1 cup (divided) reduced-sodium chicken broth
1 tbsp. cornstarch

Instructions

1. Cut the chicken into one-inch chunks.
2. Finely chop the garlic and ginger. You can substitute fresh ginger with ¼ teaspoon ground ginger. Slice lengthwise and quarter the tomatoes.
3. Use a pan over med-high heat or use a wok to warm the oil. Place the chopped breast of chicken into the pan/wok and cook three minutes.
4. Empty the soy sauce, ginger, and garlic into the pan while stirring; add the broccoli and one-half cup of the broth. Place a lid on the pan and continue cooking for two to three more minutes.
5. Mix the remainder of the broth and cornstarch until dissolved. Add it and the tomatoes to the skillet.
6. Lower the temperature to med-low. Simmer for about two minutes.

Yields: Four servings
Cal: 177.8 | P: 18.7 g | C: 22.1 g | F: 1.8 g

Chicken Creole

Ingredients
4 chicken breasts – 1-inch strips – skinless and boneless
1 cup low-sodium chili sauce
1 can (14 ounces) cut up tomatoes
¼ cup onion
½ cup celery
1 ½ cups green peppers (1 large)
2 minced garlic cloves
1 tablespoon fresh
- Basil
- Parsley
¼ teaspoon each:
- Crushed red pepper

- Salt

Instructions
1. Chop the veggies.
2. Lightly grease a pan with some cooking spray.
3. Warm the pan on the high setting. Cook the chicken for three to five minutes.
4. Lower the temperature and blend in the remainder of the fixings.
5. Once it starts to boil, cover and simmer for ten minutes.
6. Serve over a bed of rice (calories not included in counts).

Yields: One serving
Cal: 269.3| P: 32.8 g | C: 20.7 g | F: 6.3 g

Chicken Enchiladas and Sour Cream

Ingredients
½ can (14.5 ounces) each:
- Fat-free cream of chicken soup
- Mexican Rotel

1 cup fat-free sour cream
12 ounces cooked shredded chicken breast
1 tablespoon fresh chopped cilantro
½ chopped white/yellow onion
16 corn tortillas
1 cup shredded Colby/pepper jack cheese blend (reduced-fat)

Instructions
1. Mix the soup, sour cream, and cilantro in a saucepan. Heat and set to the side.
2. Grease a skillet with a small amount of oil or cooking spray. Blend the Rotel, chicken, and onions into a pan.
3. Warm the tortillas in the microwave until they are flexible.

4. Divide all of the ingredients between the tortillas and add them to the prepared dish.
5. Empty the cream sauce over the tortillas along with the rest of the cheese.
6. Bake 30 minutes at 350°F.

Yields: Eight servings (2 enchiladas each)
Cal: 252.0 | P: 18.3 g | C: 35.0 g | F: 4.5 g

Chicken Tetrazzini

Ingredients
1 tablespoon reduced calorie margarine
8 ounces sliced button mushrooms
½ cup chopped scallions – approximately 5
3 tablespoons all-purpose flour
¼ teaspoon garlic powder
Pinch of black pepper
½ pounds chicken breasts – cooked and cubed
1 cup fat-free chicken broth
¼ cup pimentos (2-ounce jar)
½ cup fat-free skim milk
2 tablespoons sherry cooking wine
8 ounces uncooked spaghetti
3 ½ tablespoons grated parmesan cheese

Instructions
1. Break the spaghetti into thirds, cook, and drain.
2. Add the margarine, scallions, and mushrooms in a pan and cook slowly for five minutes. Mix the milk, garlic powder, flour, pepper, and broth in a small container. Blend it in and continue cooking ten minutes or until thickened.
3. Add the chicken, sherry, and pimentos. Cook about two minutes.

4. Stir in the cheese and cooked spaghetti.

Yields: Six servings (one cup each)
Cal: 167 | P: 10 g | C: 25g | F: 3 g

Cola Chicken

Ingredients
3 chicken breasts
1 cup ketchup
1 can (12 ounces) diet cola
Garnish: Chopped green onion

Instructions
1. Place the breasts of chicken into a skillet and add the cola and ketchup.
2. Place a lid on the pan. Once it boils, lower the temperature setting, and continue cooking for 45 minutes.
3. Take off the lid and increase the temperature until the sauce thickens and begins to stick to the chicken.

Yields: Three servings
Cal: 193.8| P: 16.2g | C: 21.4 g | F: 1.9 g

Creamy Italian Chicken – Slow Cooker

Ingredients
2 pounds chicken breasts (no skin or bones)
½ cup water
1 can - cream of chicken soup
1 container (reduced-fat / 8 ounces) cream cheese
1 pouch - Italian dressing mix
3 cups - long grain rice – cooked – brown or white

Instructions

1. Arrange the breasts in the slow cooker. Combine the water and dressing mix. Dump it over the breasts of chicken. Put the top on the pot, and set the timer on high for four hours. If you prefer, choose the low setting for eight hours. Move the chicken to a plate.
2. In another dish, add the cream cheese and soup. Dump the mixture into the pot. Add all ingredients back into the cooker as you gently shred the chicken.
3. Continue cooking on low until all ingredients are heated.
4. Serve with the rice.

For Best Results: Use the lower setting, so all ingredients fully integrated.

Yields: Six servings (2/3 cup chicken with ½ cup of rice)
Cal: 385.4 | P: 41.0 g | C: 24.1 g | F: 12.5 g

Fifteen Minute Chili

Ingredients
½ cup chopped onions
1 pound ground turkey
1 can each of the beans (16 ounces):
- Pinto
- Kidney

1 can of (28 ounces) chopped stewed tomatoes
1 tablespoon each:
- Cumin powder
- Chili powder

½ cup salsa

Instructions

1. Rinse and drain the kidney and pinto beans.
2. Brown the turkey and onions in a large soup pot.

3. Empty the tomatoes, beans, cumin, salsa, chili powder, and garlic into the pot. Cook until boiling and serve.
4. Garnish with some cheese (count the carbs).

Yields: Four servings
Cal: 370.8 | P: 31.3 g | C: 32.3 g | F: 13.3 g

Greek Yogurt Chicken

Ingredients
4 (4 ounces each) chicken breasts
1 teaspoon garlic powder
1 cup plain Greek yogurt
½ teaspoon pepper
1 ½ teaspoons seasoning salt
½ cup grated parmesan cheese

Instructions
1. Debone and remove the skin from the chicken.
2. Set the oven temperature to 375°F.
3. Foil line a baking sheet and spray with some cooking oil.
4. Mix all of the seasonings together and coat the breasts evenly before adding to the prepared pan.
5. Bake for 45 minutes.

Yields: Four servings
Cal: 266 | P: 46 g | C: 3 g | F: 4 g

Hawaiian Turkey Burgers

Ingredients
40 ounces ground turkey
1 can (20 ounces) pineapple in unsweetened juice
2 tablespoons each:
  ▪ Minced garlic

- Ketchup

1 tablespoon each:
- Black pepper
- White vinegar

¼ teaspoon each:
- Red pepper flakes
- Salt

6 slices turkey bacon

Instructions
1. Dice the bacon into small bits and cook in a pan. Set aside in a dish. Drain and reserve the juice from the pineapple.
2. Mix the turkey, ¾ cup of the crushed pineapple, pepper, and salt in a large mixing dish.
3. In another dish, combine the ketchup, pepper flakes, pineapple juice, vinegar, and soy sauce.
4. Form the patties into 24 portions and arrange (not touching) in a baking dish. You may need two pans. Pour the pineapple juice mixture over the patties and refrigerate, covered for about an hour, turning after 30 minutes.
5. Cook the patties on a George Forman grill for two minutes or one minute on each side on a regular grill.

Yields: 24 servings
Cal: 92 | P: 9.4 g | C: 3.1 g | F: 4.1 g

Peanut Applesauce Chicken

Ingredients
1 jar (15 ounces) unsweetened applesauce
2.5 pounds - chicken pieces
½ cup powdered peanuts
¼ cup yellow mustard
1/8 cup unpacked Splenda brown sugar

To Taste: Pepper and salt

Instructions
1. Prepare the chicken in a sauté pan. When it is almost done (five minutes or so), add the powdered peanuts, sugar, mustard, and applesauce.
2. Stir and simmer over the medium heat setting on the stovetop. The internal temperature should reach 165°F.

Yields: Eight servings
Cal: 50 | P: 3 g | C: 13 g | F: 2 g

Ranch Cheddar Turkey Burgers

Ingredients
¼ cup chopped scallion
1 pound lean ground turkey
1 (one ounce) pouch dry ranch dressing mix
1 cup low-fat shredded cheese

Instructions
1. Mix all of the fixings and form six patties.
2. Cook on the grill/skillet about six to seven minutes for each side.
3. Enjoy with tomato and lettuce on a bun (not included in counts).

Yields: Six servings
Cal: 155.1 | P: 19.3 g | C: 3.6 g | F: 6.7 g

Turkey Bean Enchilada

Ingredients
2 cups white turkey meat
6 medium scallions

1 cup taco/enchilada sauce – divided
1 can of (15 ounces) pinto beans
4 tortillas – medium sized
½ cup reduced-fat shredded Mexican cheese

Instructions

1. Cook and discard any bones or fat from the turkey while cutting it into cubes.
2. Chop the green and white parts of the scallions. Drain and rinse the pinto beans.
3. Program the oven temperature in advance to 350°F.
4. Mix the beans, turkey, scallions, and ½ of the chosen sauce.
5. Fill each of the four tortillas, fold in the sides, and top/bottom.
6. Seam side down; add them to a casserole dish. Empty the remainder of the sauce on top of the enchiladas and cover with the cheese.
7. Place foil over the pan and bake about 20 minutes.

Yields: Four servings
Cal: 175 | P: 14 g | C: 19 g | F: 3 g

Thai Noodle Salad

Ingredients
6 ounces dried vermicelli
1 ½ cups shredded/chopped - cooked chicken
¼ cup each of low-sodium:
  - Vegetable broth
  - Soy sauce
½ teaspoon - crushed red peppers
2 tablespoons peanut butter
1 teaspoon each freshly minced:
  - Garlic

- Ginger

1 tablespoon fresh lime juice

3 green onions

1 sweet red pepper

Lime wedges - garnish

Instructions

1. Slice the peppers into thin strips, and diagonally slice the onions into ½-inch pieces.
2. Prepare the noodles and drain.
3. Mix in a medium saucepan: the broth, soy sauce, peanut butter, red pepper, ginger, and lime juice.
4. Blend in the pasta and toss. Add the chicken, red peppers, cilantro, and onions.
5. Garnish with the lime wedges and serve to get 100% of your daily vitamin C.

Yields: Four servings

Cal: 235.9| P: 19.4 g | C: 26 g | F: 6.6 g

Chapter 2: Seafood

Breaded Cod Fillet

Ingredients
4 (6 ounces) skinless cod
Non-stick cooking spray
¼ teaspoon black pepper
¾ teaspoon fine sea salt
3 tablespoons –divided-unsalted melted margarine
¼ cup dried whole wheat bread crumbs
Juice of 1 lemon – divided
2 tablespoons chopped chives
3 tablespoons finely chopped parsley

Instructions
1. Program the oven to 425°F.
2. Lightly coat a casserole dish with the cooking spray.
3. Flavor the cod with the pepper and salt and place in the dish.
4. Drizzle half of the lemon juice and margarine over the fish.
5. Mix the chives, parsley, and breadcrumbs in a bowl. Sprinkle it over the cod along with the remainder of lemon and margarine.
6. Bake for approximately 12 minutes.

Yields: Four servings (six ounces each)
Cal: 150 | P: 11 g | C: 6 g | F: 9 g

Crab Melt Sandwich

Ingredients
2 hard-boiled, chopped egg whites
12 ounces imitation crabmeat (coarsely chopped)
2 tablespoons chopped onion
4 tablespoons light mayonnaise
Dash of black pepper
¼ cup shredded Swiss cheese
4 slices of each:
- ¼-inch tomatoes
- Whole-wheat bread

Instructions
1. Mix the crab, egg whites, and onion, pepper, and mayonnaise.
2. Arrange the sliced of bread on the broiler pan topping with the tomatoes, crab, and mayo mixture.
3. Sprinkle each one with the Swiss cheese and broil.
- *Note*: You can use real crab but would need to adjust the counts.

Yields: Four servings
Cal: 296.3 | P: 20.3 g | C: 32.4 g | F: 9.6 g

Mock Crab Cakes

Ingredients
2 egg whites
2 pounds imitation crabmeat
1 sleeve (34) Keebler Toasteds/or other crackers – crushed
4 tablespoons light mayonnaise

Instructions
1. Program the temperature in the oven to 375°F.

2. Whisk the eggs until fluffy and blend in the mayonnaise
3. Add the crushed crackers with the eggs and combine with the crabmeat.
4. Make the patties using about ½- cup for each patty.
5. Bake 15 minutes per side.

Yields: 10 servings
Cal: 161.4 | P: 7.4 g | C: 21.6 g | F: 4.4 g

Rainbow Trout – Pan-Fried

Ingredients
8 ounces rainbow trout fillets
1 1/3 tablespoons chopped parsley
3 tablespoons yellow cornmeal
¼ teaspoon each:
  - Black pepper
  - Ground celery seeds
2 teaspoons olive oil
1 pinch salt

Instructions
1. Clean and rinse the fillets in cold water. Pat them dry.
2. Blend the pepper, cornmeal, salt, parsley, and celery to coat the fish.
3. Warm the oil in a frying pan and cook each side for two to three minutes.
4. Enjoy when they are easily flaked with a fork.

Yields: Six servings
Cal: 240 | P: 25 g | C: 10 g | F: 10 g

Salmon

BBQ Roasted Salmon

Ingredients
4 (6 ounces) salmon fillets
2 tbsp. fresh lemon juice
¼ cup pineapple juice
2 tbsp. brown sugar
½ tsp. salt
2 tsp. grated lemon rind
¾ tsp. ground cumin
4 tsp. chili powder
¼ tsp. cinnamon

Instructions
1. Program the oven temperature to 400°F.
2. Add the first three ingredients into a Ziploc plastic bag. Marinate for a minimum of one hour—turning occasionally.
3. Remove the salmon and throw the marinade in the trash.
4. Combine the rest of the ingredients and rub it over the fish.
5. Arrange them in a lightly coated baking dish for 12 to 15 minutes.
6. Garnish with some lemon.

Yields: Four servings
Cal: 225 | P: 34 g | C: 7 g | F: 6 g

Mediterranean Salmon with Pasta

Ingredients
4 (4 ounces) salmon fillets (16 ounces total)
2 medium sliced tomatoes

1 medium red bell pepper
4 cups whole wheat spaghetti - cooked
To Taste:
- Black pepper
- Lemon juice

2 tablespoons prepared pesto
Garnish: Drizzle of olive oil

Instructions

1. Slice the peppers into thin slices.
2. Program the oven setting to 400°F.
3. Arrange each of the fillets on the center of aluminum foil along with a ½ tablespoon each of the pesto sauce. Divide the veggies on/around the fish. Sprinkle with pepper and enclose the foil.
4. Bake 15 to 20 minutes.

Yields: Four servings
Cal: 407.5 | P: 38.7 g | C: 44.9 g | F: 9.2 g

Quick and Easy Salmon

Ingredients
12 ounces fresh salmon
¼ cup each soy sauce
Maple syrup/honey (not pancake syrup)
2-3 minced garlic cloves

Instructions

1. Combine all of the fixings into a Ziploc bag and shake. Place the salmon in the bag of fixings, and let it rest for a minimum of one hour in the refrigerator.
2. Mix all of the components into a baking dish and cover with a layer of aluminum foil.
3. Bake for fifteen minutes in a preheated oven at 350°F.

Yields: Four servings (3 ounces each)
Cal: 183.1 | P: 18.0 g | C: 14.9 g | F: 5.5 g

Salmon Patties

Ingredients
¼ cup green bell pepper
½ of a medium onion
1 stalk of celery
1 can of pink salmon
½ cup breadcrumbs
1 egg
½ teaspoon each:
- Chili powder
- *Optional*: Old Bay Seasoning

Instructions
1. Chop the pepper, onion, and celery into fine bits.
2. Clean the salmon by discarding the bones and skin.
3. Mix the egg, veggies, breadcrumbs, salmon, and seasonings together.
4. Scoop them out and add to a well-greased griddle.
5. Smash the patty and cook five minutes per side.
6. Top with a bit of ketchup or horseradish.

Yields: Four servings
Cal: 216.8 | P: 26 g | C: 11 g | F: 8 g

Shrimp

Creole Shrimp

Ingredients
2 teaspoons canola oil
1 chopped onion - 1 ½ cups

2 each chopped:
- Bell peppers
- Garlic cloves

3 chopped celery stalks

½ teaspoon:
- Paprika
- Thyme

¼ teaspoon:
- Cayenne pepper
- Black pepper

2 cups of each:
- Brown cooked rice
- Vegetable stock

1 cup tomato sauce – no salt added

2 tablespoons tomato paste

12 ounces peeled – deveined shrimp

Instructions
1. Using medium heat, saute the onions for two minutes. Toss in the celery and garlic and saute two more minutes; lastly, the tomato paste, spices and peppers cooking another two minutes.
2. Add the tomato sauce and stock into the pan another two minutes stirring to a boil.
3. Simmer about ten minutes and add the shrimp. Simmer two minutes.
4. Serve over rice.

Yields: 1 ¼ cup servings of Creole and ½ cup rice (four servings total)

Cal: 302.1 | P: 22.8 g | C: 45.1 g | F: 4.9 g

Lime Shrimp

Ingredients
28 large ready to cook shrimp
2 dashes salt
½ lime – juiced
2 tablespoons chopped onion
¾ teaspoon black pepper

Instructions
1. Toss all of the components into a skillet on medium heat. Toss and enjoy!

Yields: Two servings
Cal: 84.4 | P: 16.3 g | C: 2.2 g | F: 0.9 g

Shrimp Pasta

Ingredients
1 pound fresh medium shrimp
8 ounces each:
- Fettuccine
- Cream cheese (reduced-fat)

1 cup of each:
- Chicken broth
- Grated parmesan cheese

2 garlic cloves
5 ounces frozen spinach – thawed – moisture removed
To Taste: Pepper and salt

Instructions
1. Prepare the fettuccine.
2. Heat a skillet using the med-high setting. Add the chicken broth and cream cheese, stirring three to four minutes until it's well blended.

3. Add the garlic, pepper, and salt, along with the parmesan cheese.
4. Stir in the shrimp and stir until completely done. Toss in the spinach. Stir and enjoy.

Yields: Six servings
Cal: 363.5| P: 30.9g | C: 24.0 g | F: 15.2 g

Tilapia

Broiled Tilapia Parmesan

Ingredients
1 pound tilapia fillets
1 tbsp. (+) 1 ½ tsp. reduced fat mayonnaise
2 tbsp. softened butter
1/8 tsp. each of:
- Onion powder
- Ground black pepper
- Dried basil
- Celery seed
1 tbsp. fresh lemon juice

Instructions
1. Preheat the broiler on the oven. Line with foil or grease a broiling pan.
2. Combine the butter, mayonnaise, parmesan cheese, and lemon juice in a small container. Toss in the onion powder, pepper, basil, and celery salt. Stir and set to the side.
3. Place the fillets into the baking pan and broil two to three minutes. Flip them once and broil two more minutes.
4. Take the fish from the oven and coat them with the cheese mixture. Broil two more minutes.

Yields: Four servings
Cal: 177.1 | P: 19.6 g | C: 1.2 g | F: 10.5g

Lemon Garlic Tilapia

Ingredients
1 tablespoon each:
- Butter/margarine
- Olive oil

4 tilapia fillets
Juice of 1 lemon
Dash of salt
To Taste: Cayenne pepper
1 teaspoon each:
- Parsley flakes
- Garlic salt

Instructions
1. Program the oven to 400°F.
2. Place the butter in a microwavable dish along with the salt, oil, juice, parsley, and garlic powder. Saute a few minutes. Pour it over the fillets in a baking pan.
3. Sprinkle the top of the fish with the cayenne. Bake 13 minutes, and broil for another two to three minutes.

Yields: Four servings
Cal: 175.2 | P: 26.1 g | C: 1.8 g | F: 7.3 g

Oven-Fried Tilapia

Ingredients
3 egg whites
One pound (4) tilapia fillets
1 tablespoon each:
- Onion powder

- Garlic powder
- Grated parmesan cheese
- Cajun seasoning

1 ½ cups finely ground Fiber One cereal/oven-fry bread
Non-stick cooking spray

Instructions
1. Program the oven temperature to 400°F.
2. Whisk the egg whites until frothy.
3. In a separate container, combine all of the seasonings, cheese, and cereal.
4. Lightly spray a cookie sheet and add the fish. Spritz a small amount of oil directly on the fish.
5. Bake 8 to 10 minutes.

Yields: Four servings (4 ounces each)
Cal: 184.7 | P: 27.9 g | C: 22.1 g | F: 3.1 g

Tuna

Best Ever Tuna Salad

Ingredients
2/3 cup cottage cheese (non-fat)
1 can of albacore tuna
4 tablespoons plain low-fat yogurt
1 stalk of celery
¼ small onion
1 teaspoon Dijon mustard
Pinch of dill
Splash lemon juice

Instructions
1. Finely chop the onion and celery.

2. Get a big dish for two and have lunch with all of the goodies in a bowl. (Of course, make them even servings.)

Yields: Two servings
Cal: 190.3 | P: 32.5 g | C: 11.7 g | F: 2.2 g

Crunchy Tuna Patties

Ingredients
4 egg whites
4 cans (3 ounces) tuna packed in water
¼ cup each:
- Chopped water chestnuts/diced red pepper/capers
- Grated carrot

16 crushed Wheat Thin crackers
1 tablespoon minced onion
To Taste
- Dried mustard
- Dill
- Pepper

Instructions
1. Combine all of the fixings and form eight patties.
2. Use cooking oil to spray a skillet. Over medium temperature on the stovetop, brown the patties two to three minutes for each side.

Yields: Eight servings
Cal: 80 | P: 12 g | C: 4 g | F: 1 g

Tuna and White Bean Salad

Ingredients
1 can of (15.5 ounces) chickpeas/white beans
2 cans tuna (chunk light in water)

1 red bell pepper
¼ cup onion
Juice of 1 lemon
1 tablespoon olive oil
Optional

- Spinach
- Tomatoes
- Parsley

Instructions

1. Drain and rinse the beans. Drain the tuna. Dice the onion and pepper.
2. Combine all of the goodies and chill for a minimum of four hours.
3. Serve over a bed of greens.

Yields: Four servings
Cal: 193.2 | P: 22.6 g | C: 20.4 | F: 4.3 g

Chapter 3: Soups

Barley and Beef Soup

Ingredients
1 pound beef – stew meat/chuck/steak
1 tablespoon butter
½ cup each chopped:
- Carrots
- Onions
- Celery

4 cups each:
- Water
- Beef broth

¾ cup barley (quick-cook)
1 teaspoon each:
- Salt
- Black pepper

½ teaspoon each:
- Oregano
- Basil

1 can of (14.5 ounces) diced tomatoes

Instructions
1. Put the butter in a soup kettle and saute the celery, carrot, and onion for about five minutes.
2. Pour in the water, broth, tomatoes, beef, pepper, salt, barley, basil, and oregano. When it begins to boil, lower the temperature and cook about twenty minutes to an hour depending on how you like its consistency.

Yields: 12servings
Cal: 198.6 | P: 13.7 g | C: 16.3 g | F: 8.7 g

Cabbage Vegetable Soup

Ingredients
1 medium diced onion
1 can each:
- 28 ounces - crushed tomatoes
- 14.5 ounces green beans
- 15 ounces can pinto beans
- 12 ounces sweet yellow corn

3 medium diced carrots
1 head shredded cabbage
3 diced stalks of celery

Instructions
1. Pour the tomatoes, cabbage, celery, onion, and carrots in a pot. Simmer about 20 minutes over medium heat.
2. Add the canned veggies and serve.

Yields: Six servings (1 ½ cups each)
Cal: 165.2 | P: 8.3 g | C: 36.6 g | F: 1.8 g

Chicken Taco Stew – Slow Cooker

Ingredients
2 chicken breasts – no bones or skin
2 cans diced tomatoes w/chilies (14 ½ oz. each)
1 chopped onion
1 can tomato sauce (8 oz.)
1 can corn (16 oz.)
1 can each of 16 oz. beans:
- Kidney
- Black

1 package of taco seasoning (1.25 ounces)

Instructions

1. Mix all of the fixings except for the chicken in the crock pot.
2. Arrange the breasts on top and cover with the lid.
3. Cook on the high setting for three to four hours. If you prefer, you can choose the low setting for six to eight hours.
4. Shred the chicken about 30 minutes before you are ready to serve.
5. Blend it back into the soup pot and heat until you are ready to eat.

Yields: 14 servings – 1 cup each
Cal: 158.7| P: 14 g | C: 24.4 g | F: 1.1 g

Chicken Tortilla Soup – Slow Cooker

Ingredients
1 lb. frozen chicken
1 medium chopped onion
1 can of:
- Whole peeled tomatoes (15 oz.)
- Enchilada sauce (10 oz.)
- Chopped green chile peppers (4 oz.)
- Black beans – rinsed (15 oz.)
3 cans (14.5 oz. each) chicken broth
1 pkg. frozen corn (10 oz.)
1 teaspoon cumin
2 minced garlic cloves
¼ teaspoon black pepper

Instructions

1. Arrange the chicken, enchilada sauce, tomatoes, green chiles, onions, and garlic into the crock pot.

2. Flavor the pot fixings with the pepper, salt, and cumin. Empty the chicken broth, black beans, and corn. Cook low for six to eight hrs. or high for three hrs.
3. Garnish with some shredded cheese, avocados, sour cream or other ingredients of your choosing. Be sure to add the additional calories.

Yields: Eight servings
Cal: 169.1 | P: 17.4 g | C: 20.3 g | F: 2.5 g

Corn Chowder Soup

Ingredients
1 tablespoon olive oil
1 package frozen whole kernel corn (10 ounces)
2 tbsp. each finely diced:
- Green pepper
- Onion
- Celery
- Chopped fresh parsley
1 cup each of:
- Peeled – diced potatoes
- Water
Pepper if desired
¼ teaspoon each:
- Salt
- Paprika
2 cups low-fat/skim milk
¼ cup minced fresh parsley
2 tablespoons flour

Instructions
1. Pour the oil into a skillet on the stovetop using the medium heat setting. Also, add the celery, onion, and green peppers into a pan and saute for two minutes.

2. Blend in the potatoes, corn, pepper, salt, water, and paprika. Let it boil and lower the temperature to the medium setting and continue cooking for ten minutes.
3. Mix the flour in a jar with a ½ cup of milk, and shake. Blend it in with the cooked veggies along with the rest of the milk.
4. Cook until it thickens and garnish with parsley.

Yields: Four – 1 cup servings
Cal: 202.5 | P: 8.0 g | C: 32.7 g | F: 5.3 g

Curried Carrot Soup

Ingredients
½ pound chopped carrots
½ tbsp. of olive oil (extra-virgin)
1 garlic clove
1 tsp. curry powder
¼-inch piece fresh mashed ginger
3 cups vegetable broth – low sodium
¼ cup light coconut milk

Instructions
1. Add the oil to a skillet on the stovetop using the high heat setting. Toss in the garlic, ginger, curry powder, carrots, and 1 ½ cups of the vegetable broth.
2. When it begins to boil, reduce the temperature, and cook until the carrots are soft (15 to 20 minutes). Pour in the remainder of the vegetable broth.
3. Puree the mixture in the blender when they are mushy and have cooled.
4. Add the puree back into the pot and heat on medium high, pouring in the milk.
5. Serve warm and enjoy with a sprinkle of freshly cracked black pepper.

Yields: Four servings
Cal: 63.4 | P: 0.7 g | C: 8.4 g | F: 2.9 g

15-Minute Chili

Ingredients
½ cup chopped onions
1 lb. ground turkey
1 can chopped stewed tomatoes (28 ounces)
1 can (16 ounces) each:
- Pinto beans
- Kidney beans
1 tablespoon each:
- Cumin powder
- Chili powder
½ cup salsa

Instructions
1. Wash and drain the kidney and pinto beans.
2. Brown the onions and turkey in a large pot.
3. Empty the tomatoes, beans, cumin, salsa, chili powder, and garlic into the pot. Cook until boiling and serve.
4. Garnish with some cheese (count the carbs).

Yields: Four servings
Cal: 370.8 | P: 31.3 g | C: 32.3 g | F: 13.3 g

5 Ingredient Soup

Ingredients
1 can each of (14.4 ounces):
Corn
Fat-free chicken broth
Diced tomatoes (no-salt added)
Black beans
Fat-free refried beans

Instructions

1. Wash and completely drain the corn and black beans. In a medium saucepan, mix all of the fixings using a whisk to blend in the refried beans.
2. Simmer and serve.
3. Garnish with some avocado, green onions, or sour cream.

Yields: Ten servings
Cal: 128.0 | P: 7.3 g | C: 24.9 g | F: 0.6 g

French Onion Soup

Ingredients
1 medium yellow onion
¼ cup water
4 cups beef broth
½ cup part-skim mozzarella cheese – shredded
2 slices whole-wheat bread/2 tablespoons croutons

Instructions

1. Toss the diced onions into the pot of the boiling water and continue cooking until the onions are shining. Pour in the beef broth and continue cooking for another 15 to 20 minutes
2. When it's done, add two cups into a dish. Garnish each one with one ounce of shredded mozzarella and a slice of bread or substitute 1 tablespoon of croutons.
3. Place it under the broiler and melt the cheese, if you like it that way.

Yields: Two servings
Cal: 165.9 | P: 14.6 g | C: 14.7 g | F: 6.1 g

Fully Loaded Potato Soup

Ingredients
3 large sliced carrots
6 large cubed potatoes
3 chopped celery stalks
2 chopped onions
4 chicken bouillon cubes
1 can - non-fat evaporated milk
6 cups of water
Optional: Shredded cheddar cheese (not in counts)

Instructions
1. Combine the veggies, water, and bouillon in a large slow cooker.
2. Cook on the high setting for three to four hours or the low for eight to ten hours.
3. Once the time has elapsed, add the milk and heat.
4. Serve and enjoy.

Yields: Twelve servings
Cal: 170.7 | P: 5.9 g | C: 36.7 g | F: 0.4 g

Southwestern Chicken Soup

Ingredients
1 pound chicken breasts (16 ounces) bite-sized pieces
1 small chopped onion
1 jalapeno pepper –chopped
3 chopped garlic cloves
4 cups fresh spinach /4 ounces frozen
1 chopped green pepper
1 tablespoon each:
- Olive oil
- Cumin

2 chopped avocados
1 can (14 ounces) each:

- Low-sodium chopped tomatoes
- Pinto/black beans – drained and rinsed

¼ cup cilantro – torn
2 limes – juiced
2 cups cooked brown rice
1-quart chicken stock

Instructions

1. Prepare the rice and heat the oil using the medium heat setting on the stovetop. Toss in garlic, onions, and peppers. Cook approximately five minutes.
2. Lower the temperature setting to medium and add the tomatoes. Simmer about ten minutes.
3. Take the pan off of the burner and blend in the lime juice, mixing well. Add salt and pepper if desired.
4. Add ½ cup of rice to each bowl and garnish with a sprinkle of avocado and cilantro.

Note: Leave the seeds in the jalapeno for more spice.
Yields: 8 (one cup servings)
Cal: 270.5 | P: 19.8 g | C: 25.8 g | F: 10.6 g

Thai Chicken Coconut Soup

Ingredients
12 ounces breast of chicken
1 cup coconut milk
1 cup quartered white mushrooms
5 ginger slices - fresh and peeled
1 ½ cups chicken broth/stock
1 teaspoon Thai chili paste
1 lemon
4 sliced green onions

1 tablespoon shredded basil
Pinch of white pepper

Instructions
1. Discard any skin and bones from the chicken breasts, and cover with water in a small pan until it just starts to boil. Poach it for 15 minutes or until the internal temperature reads 165°F.
2. In another pan, prepare the stock, coconut milk, ginger, white part of the green onion, and mushrooms. Simmer for ten minutes after you add the chili paste.
3. Slice the chicken into chunks and toss into the soup. Blend in the lemon juice, along with the pepper and basil.
4. Garnish with some chopped green onion.

Yields: Four servings
Cal: 141.5 | P: 22.7g | C: 6.4 g | F: 3.6 g

Tomato Soup

Ingredients
1 cup chopped yellow/white onion
3 minced garlic cloves
2 tbsp. olive oil
2 pounds tomatoes
½ tsp. dried thyme
1 tbsp. brown sugar
¼ tsp. red pepper flakes
4 small slices of bread
1 tbsp. balsamic vinegar
1 ½ cups chicken/vegetable stock (low-sodium)

Instructions
1. Discard the seeds and dice the tomatoes. Remove the crust from the bread.

2. Pour the oil into a stock pot along with the onions and garlic. Saute five minutes.
3. Blend in the tomatoes, thyme, sugar, pepper, and bread. Cook for three minutes.
4. Puree with a food processor/immersion blender.
5. Pour the stock in slowly, and simmer for ten minutes. Lastly, pour in the vinegar and cook approximately two additional minutes.

Yields: Eight servings
Cal: 98.9 | P: 2.5 g | F: 4.1 g | C: 14.3 g

Vegetable Curry – Slow Cooker

Ingredients
1 tablespoon canola oil
4 medium carrots (2 cups)
1 thinly sliced onion
3 garlic cloves- thinly sliced
1 teaspoon ground cumin
2 tablespoons curry powder
½ teaspoon each:
  ▪ Turmeric
  ▪ Garam masala
8 ounces fresh/frozen green beans
4-5 potatoes – quartered
1 cup/2 large diced tomatoes
3 cups chickpeas (canned- drained-rinsed)
2 cups vegetable stock
½ cup each:
  ▪ Frozen peas
  ▪ Light coconut milk

Instructions
1. Slice the carrots about 1/3 inches thick.

2. Warm the oil and add the carrots and onions, sautéing for about three to four minutes. Add the cumin, curry powder, garlic, turmeric, and garam masala to the pan and cook two more minutes.
3. Transfer the veggies to the slow cooker. Add the green beans, potatoes, chickpeas, and vegetable stock to the cooker.
4. Set the timer for 5 ½ hours on the low setting. After that time elapses, add the peas and milk cooking 15 more minutes.

Yields: Eight servings (one cup each)
Cal: 183.6 | P: 7 g | C: 30.5 g | F: 3.8 g

Vegetarian Chili

Ingredients
1 can (15 oz.) each:
- Pinto beans
- Black beans
- Light red kidney beans
- Dark red kidney beans

1 can (28 oz.) diced tomatoes
2 cans (28 oz.) crushed tomatoes
3 cups celery
1 medium red onion
1 small diced each of bell pepper:
- Red
- Yellow

4 tbsp. chili powder
3 tbsp. garlic powder
2 tbsp. ground cumin

Instructions
1. Drain and rinse all of the beans. Dice the veggies.
2. On the stove top using the medium temperature setting, lightly spray the pan and cook the veggies about six to seven minutes.
3. Mix the spices, beans, and tomatoes in a slow cooker (6-7 hours on low) or a Dutch oven (3-4 hours on high).
4. Heat and enjoy.

Yields: Eight servings
Cal: 279.8 | P: 14.7 g | C: 58.4 g | F: 2.2 g

White Chicken Chili

Ingredients
2 pounds chicken breasts (boneless – skinless)
3 grated garlic cloves
½ tsp. chili powder
1 tbsp. olive oil
1 diced onion
1 teaspoon each:
- Salt
- Cumin

1/8 tsp. each:
- Ground cloves
- Cayenne pepper

4 cans cannellini/ white kidney beans (15.5 ounces)
1 can of low-sodium chicken stock (28 ounces)
2 cans green chilis (4 ounces)
2 cups frozen corn
1 lime
¾ cup low-fat Monterey jack cheese

Instructions

1. Cut the chicken into one-inch chunks. Drain and rinse the beans.
2. Use the medium heat setting on the stovetop and pour in the oil, onion, and chicken. Cook for about five to seven minutes.
3. Toss in the grated cloves of garlic along with the spices, cooking for an additional one to two minutes.
4. Pour in the stock and beans, and simmer twenty-five minutes. Blend in the chilies and corn, and cook about five more minutes.
5. Take it away from the heat and squeeze the lime juices into the chili.
6. Add one tablespoon of cheese for each cup of soup.

Yields: 12 servings
Cal: 234.5 | P: 25.0 g | C: 20.2 g | F: 6.3 g

Chapter 4: Pork

Asian Pork Tenderloin

Ingredients
2 tablespoons each:
- Rice vinegar
- Worcestershire sauce
- Lemon juice

1/3 cup each of:
- Brown sugar
- Light soy sauce

1 tablespoon each of:
- Ginger
- Dry mustard

1 ½ teaspoons pepper
4 minced garlic cloves
2 lbs. pork tenderloin

Instructions
1. Program the oven to 375°F.
2. Add all of the ingredients into a freezer bag along with the tenderloin.
3. Place in the fridge overnight.
4. When ready to cook, bake for 30 to 40 minutes.
5. *Note*: You can also use the slow cooker for four to six hours.

Yields: Eight servings (4 ounces each)
Cal: 256 | P: 34 g | C: 9 g | F: 9 g

Balsamic-Glazed Pork Tenderloin

Ingredients
1 ½ - pounds pork tenderloin
¼ tsp. salt
1/8 tsp. black pepper
3 tbsp. brown sugar blend Splenda
¼ cup balsamic vinegar

Instructions
1. Set the oven temperature to 425°F.
2. Use cold water to rinse the pork, patting it dry. Flavor it if desired with the pepper and salt. Arrange the tenderloin in a skillet to brown all sides until caramelized.
3. Take the pork from the pan, using med-low and add the vinegar to loosen the browned bits. Toss in the brown sugar and add the pork back into the pan.
4. Bake for 25 minutes.

Yields: Six servings – four ounces each
Cal: 257.4| P: 33.3 g | C: 7.4 g | F: 9.3 g

BBQ Pulled Pork Roast – Slow Cooker

Ingredients
1 cup each of:
- Chopped onions
- Chopped celery
- Water
- Barbecue sauce
- Ketchup

2 tablespoons each:
- Worcestershire sauce
- Vinegar
- Brown sugar

1 teaspoon each:

- Salt
- Chili powder

½ teaspoon each:
- Garlic powder
- Pepper

3 pounds boneless pork roast

Instructions
1. Mix all of the ingredients in the slow cooker.
2. Arrange the roast in the pot last.
3. Place the lid on the cooker and set the timer for six to seven hours on the high setting.
4. Transfer the meat to a platter, shred, and return to the pot.
5. Simmer until hot and enjoy.

Yields: 12 servings
Cal: 296.9 | P: 32.4 g | C: 12.3 g | F: 11.9 g

Cocoa Pork Tenderloin

Ingredients
1 tsp. instant coffee
½ tsp. each:
- Cinnamon
- Chili powder

1 tbsp. each
- Cocoa powder – unsweetened
- Canola Oil

1 lb. pork tenderloin

Instructions
1. Trim the fat from the pork as well as the white tendon. Combine the spices.

2. Rub the meat with the oil and spices. Add the tenderloin to a heavy-duty iron skillet and sear the meat on high heat.
3. Place in the oven for 15 minutes (internal temperature of 145°F).
4. Remove the pan and arrange the meat on a cutting board to rest five minutes. Slice and serve.

Yields: Four servings
Cal: 264 | P: 33.7 g | Carbs: 1.2 g | Fat: 13.1 g

Grilled Honey Garlic Pork Chops

Ingredients
3 tablespoons soy sauce
¼ (+) 1/8 cup honey
6 boneless fat-free pork loin chops
6 minced garlic cloves

Instructions
1. Blend the soy sauce, garlic, and honey. Evenly cover the chops.
2. Save the honey mix for basting.
3. Grill over med-high heat with a closed lid.

Yields: Six servings
Cal: 204.3 | P: 19.9 g | C: 18.4 g | F: 5.7 g

Mango Curried Pork Chops

4 (4-ounces) boneless pork chops – ¾-inch thick
¼ cup raisins
1 tsp. cornstarch
2 tsp. curry powder
¼ tsp. seasoned salt

4 green sliced onions
1/3 cup chicken broth
2 tsp. vegetable oil
2 tbsp. flaked coconut
1 fresh mango

Instructions
1. Peel and dice the mango.
2. Sprinkle the chops with the seasoned salt and curry powder.
3. Warm the oil in a skillet and brown the chops. Cook for about eight minutes. Flip one time only.
4. Take the chops from the skillet, and save the juices.
5. In a small mixing dish, blend the chicken broth and cornstarch. Toss in the raisins, onions, and broth mixture into the skillet – cooking until slightly thickened.
6. Transfer the chops back into the skillet and heat.
7. Garnish with the mango and coconut.

Yields: One serving
Cal: 274.6| P: 24.6 g | C: 19.9g | F: 11.1 g

Mustard Brown Sugar Pork Chops

Ingredients
1/3 cup yellow mustard
½ cup brown sugar
6 boneless pork loin chops

Instructions
1. Blend the sugar and mustard together and pour over the chops.
2. Bake 25 minutes at 350°F.

Yields: Six servings

Cal: 228.1| P: 20.7 g | C: 24.6 g | F: 7.8 g

Pork with Greens and Beans – Slow Cooker

Ingredients for the Spice Rub:
2 pounds pork shoulder
1 tablespoon chili powder
½ teaspoon each:
- Kosher or sea salt
- Red pepper flakes

3 halved garlic cloves
1 cup chicken stock (low-sodium)
2 cups kale/escarole – chopped
14.5-ounce cans each of:
- 1 low-sodium diced tomatoes
- 2 cans cannellini beans

½ cup pepitas/pumpkin seeds

Instructions
1. Remove all fat pockets.
2. *Prepare the rub:* Mix the salt, pepper, and chili powder. Rub it on the meat the night before/at least one hour before cooking. Refrigerate.
3. Arrange the pork in the crockpot along with the garlic. Pour the stock over the meat. Cook five to six hours.
4. Take the lid off, break up the meat into chunks. Blend in the kale, beans, and tomatoes – cooking another hour.
5. In a dry skillet, toast the pepitas.

Yields: Eight servings (one-cup serving (+) 1 tablespoon of pepitas as garnish)
Cal: 285.9 | P: 25.9g | C: 11.7 g | F: 15.6

Sweet & Sour Pork

Ingredients
1 can (15 ounces) unsweetened pineapple chunks
1 lb. lean pork tenderloin
¼ cup Splenda brown sugar blend
1 tbsp. low-sodium soy sauce
½ cup water
2 tbsp. cornstarch
½ teaspoon salt
2 medium sliced green peppers
1 small onion
1/3 cup wine vinegar
3 cups cooked brown rice

Instructions
1. Cut the pork into thin strips.
2. On the stovetop, cook the pork until done. Drain the fat from the skillet.
3. Drain and reserve the juice from the pineapple.
4. Mix the vinegar, water, cornstarch, sugar, salt, pineapple juice, and soy sauce in a small dish and add to the skillet. Let it cook about two minutes for the sauce to thicken.
5. Add the pork and cook on the low setting about 30 minutes. Blend in the pineapple, peppers, and onion. Cook about five more minutes.
6. Enjoy over the rice.

Yields: Six servings
Cal: 248 | P: 18 g | C: 36 g | F: 3.5 g

Chapter 5: Beef

Bavarian Beef

Ingredients
1 tablespoon olive oil
1 bay leaf
1 ¼ pounds stewing beef
½ small head of cabbage
1 large onion
¾ teaspoon caraway seeds
Pinch of black pepper and salt
1 tablespoon sugar
1 ½ - cups water
¼ cup cider/white vinegar
¼ cup crushed gingersnaps

Instructions
1. Cut the beef into 1-inch chunks. Thinly slice the onion. Cut the cabbage into four wedges.
2. Brown the beef in a skillet using the oil. Remove and drain the meat. Cook the onion in the same pan for about five minutes and add the meat back into the skillet.
3. Pour in the water, bay leaf, pepper, salt, and caraway seeds.
4. Once the mixture begins to boil, lower the temperature, and simmer for one hour and fifteen minutes.
5. Mix in the sugar and vinegar. Stir and add the cabbage on top of the meat. Simmer the ingredients covered for another 45 minutes.
6. Transfer the cabbage and meat to a platter.
7. Strain the drippings and add enough water to make one cup of liquid. Blend in the gingersnaps to the pan, cooking until thickened.
8. Serve the sauce over the meat and veggies.

Yields: Five servings (5 ounces each portion)
Cal: 256.1 | P: 29.1 g | C: 12.1 g | F: 10.1 g

BBQ Steak/Chicken Wrap

Ingredients
8 ounces sliced - cooked steak/chicken breast
2 cups baby spinach
4 (8-inch) whole wheat fat-free tortillas
1 cup of each:
- Frozen – thawed corn
- Can black beans

½ cup shredded cheese (low-fat cheddar)
¼ cup barbecue sauce

Instructions
1. Rinse and drain the beans.
2. Preheat the oven to 400F. Lightly spray a baking dish.
3. Prepare and roll up each of the wraps and heat thoroughly for ten minutes.

Yields: Four servings
Cal: 405.5 | P: 31.5 g | C: 45.1 g | F: 11.4 g

Beef and Mushroom- Slow Cooker

Ingredients
1 pound lean stewing beef
1 can of mushroom soup (creamy, low-fat)
½ cup water
1 pouch of dry onion soup mix
8 ounces fresh sliced/whole mushrooms

Instructions

1. Use the medium heat setting to lightly brown the meat in a frying pan. Add it to the slow cooker (4 quart is best).
2. Add the meat to the bottom and the mushrooms. Combine the soup mix water, along with the can of soup together and empty into the pot.
3. Serve over some noodles or brown rice. (Count the calories.)

Yields: Four servings
Cal: 410.5| P: 34.8 g | C: 12.4 g | F: 23.9 g

Buffalo Chicken Sandwich

Ingredients
2 skinless chicken breasts (4 ounces each)
¼ cup each:
- Hot sauce
- Breadcrumbs

Pepper and salt to taste
1 tablespoon each:
- Vinegar
- Butter

Tomato and lettuce
2 whole grain hamburger buns

Instructions

1. Set the oven temperature to 450°F.
2. Combine the pepper, salt, and breadcrumbs.
3. Pound the meat with a mallet between some plastic to flatten it for even cooking.
4. Use the breadcrumbs to cover the entire chicken and arrange it on a lightly sprayed casserole dish. Cook in the oven for 25 to 30 minutes.

5. In a plastic bag, add the butter, vinegar, and hot sauce along with the chicken. Shake to coat it evenly and add to the toasted buns.
6. Add the tomatoes and lettuce.
7. Add the extra calories if you add some dressing or mayo.

Yields: Two servings
Cal: 268.7 | P: 18.1 g | C: 34.3 g | F: 8.7 g

Diet Coke Sloppy Joes

Ingredients
16 ounces ground beef
1 cup diet cola
2 tablespoons each:
- Dry mustard
- White vinegar

1 tablespoon Worcestershire sauce
Garlic powder

Instructions
1. Brown the beef in a skillet, drain and place it back into the pan.
2. Add the remainder of the fixings and stir.
3. Cook uncovered on the low setting for 30 minutes.

Yields: Four servings
Cal: 162.5| P: 24.0g | C: 2.5 g | F: 4.5 g

Ginger Beef

Ingredients
2 tablespoons each:
- Lite soy sauce
- Seasoned rice vinegar

2 teaspoons each:

- Cornstarch
- Ground ginger

½ cup water

1 teaspoon garlic powder

10 slices fresh ginger root (1-inch diameter)

8 large scallions

1 pound flank steak

Instructions

1. Slice the ginger into wafer thin slices, and dice. Wash and slice the scallions.
2. Mix the garlic powder, ginger, water, soy sauce, and vinegar.
3. Slice the meat into one-inch strips against the grain of the meat. Chill in the fridge for about 20 minutes.
4. Spray a skillet/wok with non-stick cooking oil. Using the high setting, add the veggies and meat. It should take about ten minutes to brown.
5. At the end of the cooking cycle; mix the cornstarch with some water and stir quickly into the juices to thicken.

Yields: Four servings

Cal: 207.6| P: 22.9 g | C: 10.3 g | F: 8.0 g

Ground Beef Casserole - Keema

Ingredients

1 ½ pounds lean ground sirloin

1 cup of each:

- Diced potatoes
- Chopped onions
- Frozen peas

1 tablespoon curry powder

2 cups crushed tomatoes

½ teaspoon each:
- Ginger
- Turmeric
- Cinnamon

Salt and pepper - if desired

Instructions
1. Brown the onions and sirloin in a pan. Add the potatoes, peas, tomatoes, and spices.
2. Simmer for 25 minutes adding a pinch of pepper and salt.
3. It should look have the consistency similar to chili.

Yields: Six servings
Cal: 197.3 | P: 22.4 g | C: 11.6 g | F: 7.0 g

Ground Beef and Potato Casserole

Ingredients
1 pound lean ground beef
¼ cup water mixed with soup
1 can cream of mushroom soup (10.75 ounces - Campbell's Healthy Quest)
1 cup chopped onions
3-4 medium potatoes
¼ teaspoon each:
- Black pepper
- Salt (optional)

Instructions
1. Program the oven to 350°F.
2. Prepare the potatoes thinly sliced with skins.
3. Brown the onions and beef; drain.
4. In a 9x11-inch (2 quarts) casserole dish, lightly spray and add a layer of potatoes with a layer of beef.

5. Pour ½ of the soup mixture over this and add an additional layer with the rest of the ingredients.
6. Bake one hour.

Yields: Six to eight servings
Cal: 166.3 | P: 14.0 g | C: 18.5 g | F: 4.1 g

Lasagna in the Skillet

Ingredients
3 minced garlic cloves
1 small chopped onion
1 pound lean ground beef
1 can each:
- 8 ounces tomato sauce
- 14 ounces diced tomatoes

1 ¼ - cups water
2 ½ - cups broken whole wheat lasagna noodles
1 teaspoon each:
- Oregano leaves
- Salt
- Basil leaves
- Parsley flakes

1 cup cottage cheese (fat-free)
¼ cup grated parmesan cheese (fat-free)
1 egg
Optional: Pepper and dried basil
Garnish: Shredded mozzarella cheese

Instructions
1. Brown the garlic, onions, and beef in a large skillet. Drain and add the tomatoes, sauce, water, salt, oregano, basil, and parsley. Stir, add the noodles and bring to boiling.
2. Reduce the heat and continue cooking slowly in the skillet covered for twenty minutes.

3. Blend in the Parmesan and cottage cheese along with the egg.
4. Sprinkle with the pepper and basil.
5. Arrange a rounded tablespoon of the cheese mix onto the pasta.
6. Place a lid on the pot and cook five minutes. Sprinkle with the mozzarella and enjoy.

Yields: Six servings
Cal: 342.3 | P: 28 g | C: 34.5 g | F: 10.7 g

Meatloaf Muffins

Ingredients
1 cup stewed tomatoes
1 pound lean ground beef
4 tablespoons ketchup
2 tablespoons - heavy whipping cream
1 cup dried bread crumbs
1 jumbo egg
1 teaspoon salt
3 teaspoons Worcestershire sauce
1 tablespoon each:
  ▪ Cider vinegar
  ▪ Black pepper
6 teaspoons brown sugar

Instructions
1. Combine all ingredients – omit brown sugar, cider, and ketchup.
2. Fill the 12 muffin tins.
3. Combine the ketchup, cider, and brown sugar in a small dish to spoon over each muffin.
4. Bake 30 minutes at 350°F.

Yields: 12 servings
Cal: 176.7 | P: 9.1 g | C: 12.6 g | F: 9.9 g

Mushroom and Beef - Slow Cooker

Ingredients
1 pound lean stewing beef
1 package onion soup mix - dry
1 can cream of mushroom soup (low-fat)
½ cup water
8 ounces fresh sliced/whole mushrooms

Instructions
1. Use the medium heat setting to cook the beef in a skillet and add it to the slow cooker (four- quart size is best).
2. Add the meat on the bottom and the mushrooms. Mix the soup, water, and pour into the pot.
3. Serve over some noodles or brown rice. (Count the calories.)

Yields: Four servings
Cal: 410.5| P: 34.8 g | F: 23.9 g | C: 12.4 g

Slimmer Beef Stroganoff - Stir Fry

Ingredients
1 ½ - cups whole wheat bow tie pasta
1 pound beef tenderloin tips
1/3 cup chopped onion
½ pound sliced mushrooms
2 teaspoons olive oil
1 can (10.5 ounces) beef broth
2 tablespoons whole wheat flour

Instructions

1. Prepare the pasta.
2. Cut the beef into one-inch cubes and trim away all fat.
3. Lightly grease a pan with some non-stick cooking spray. Use the medium heat setting on the stovetop and add the beef. Stir fry for three to five minutes. Transfer to a dish.
4. In the same pan add the oil, onions, and mushrooms. Cook for two to three minutes.
5. Blend in the flour and broth stirring until mixed.
6. Once it begins to boil, cook for about two minutes. Add pepper and salt.

Yields: One serving
Cal: 514.5| P: 30.9 g | C: 42.4 g | F: 24.1 g

Chapter 6: Veggies and Fruits

Acorn Squash- Stuffed with Cheese

Ingredients
1 pound ground turkey breast (extra-lean)
2 acorn squash
1 can (8 ounces) tomato sauce
1 cup each:
- Sliced fresh mushrooms
- Chopped onion
- Diced celery

1 teaspoon each:
- Garlic powder
- Basil
- Oregano

1 pinch black pepper
1/8 teaspoon salt
1 cup shredded cheddar cheese (reduced-fat)

Instructions
1. Program the oven temperature to 350°F.
2. Slice the squash in half and remove the seeds. Arrange the squash, cut side down, in a dish and microwave on high for 20 minutes.
3. Brown the turkey in a skillet and add the onion and celery. Saute two to three minutes. Blend in the mushrooms, and add the sauce and seasonings. Divide into quarters and spoon into the squash.
4. Cover and bake for 15 minutes.
5. Garnish with the cheese and bake until the cheese has melted.

Yields: Four servings
Cal: 299 | P: 30 g | F: 4 g | C: 38 g

Baked Tomatoes

Ingredients
Olive oil spray
5-6 large tomatoes
Greek seasoning
¼ cup low-fat parmesan cheese
Optional: ¼ cup pine nuts

Instructions
1. Set the oven temperature in advance to 350°F. Spray a baking pan with the olive oil.
2. Slice the tomatoes lengthwise into halves and arrange them on the baking pan.
3. Sprinkle them with the cheese, nuts, and a bit of Greek seasoning as you desire.
4. Bake on the middle oven rack for 50 minutes.

Yields: Six servings
Cal: 73| P: 3 g | C: 6 g | F: 5 g

Black Bean and Rice Casserole

Ingredients
1 cup vegetable broth
1/3 cup each:
   ▪ Diced onion
   ▪ Brown rice
1 tablespoon olive oil
1 lb. chopped chicken breast (no skin or bones)
1 medium thinly sliced zucchini
½ cup sliced mushrooms

¼ teaspoon cayenne pepper
½ teaspoon cumin
1/3 cup shredded carrots
1 can (4 ounces) diced green chilies
1 can (15 ounces) drained black beans
2 cups shredded Swiss cheese

Instructions
1. Prepare a pot with the vegetable broth and rice, bringing it to a boil. Lower the heat setting and cook covered on low for 45 minutes.
2. Program the oven temperature to 350°F.
3. Spray a baking dish with some cooking spray.
4. Pour the oil in a pan over medium heat. Toss in the onion and cook until tender, and blend in the chicken, zucchini, mushrooms, and seasonings. Continue cooking until the chicken is heated and the zucchini is lightly browned.
5. In a large mixing dish, combine the onion, cooked rice, chicken, zucchini, beans, chilies, mushrooms, one cup of Swiss cheese, and the carrots.
6. Empty the ingredients into the casserole dish along with the remainder of the Swiss cheese as a topping. Cover and bake 30 minutes. Uncover, and continue cooking ten more minutes.

Yields: Eight servings
Cal: 267| P: 31 g | C: 22 g | F: 6 g

Broccoli Casserole

Ingredients
4 cups cut up broccoli
1 sleeve Ritz crackers
2 cups cheddar cheese

Instructions
1. Add the casserole ingredients into a Pyrex dish with the crumbled crackers on top.
2. Bake long enough to melt the cheese at 375°F.

Yields: 12 servings
Cal: 90.5 | P: 10.3 g | C: 9.8 g | F: 2.3 g

Chickpea and Feta Salad

Ingredients
¾ cup chopped raw vegetables
¼ cup each:
- Can/fresh chickpeas
- Crumbled feta cheese

1 tablespoon lemon juice
2 tablespoons olive oil
1 teaspoon dried oregano
Dash each of:
- Pepper
- Salt

Instructions
1. Use your imagination for the chopped veggies. Include peppers, avocado, tomatoes, onions, and celery or your favorites.
2. Rinse and drain the chickpeas.
3. Combine all of the ingredients and chill in the fridge until ready to serve.

Yields: One serving
Cal: 285.2 | P: 10.2 g | C: 22.2 g | F: 18.4 g

Coleslaw

Ingredients
1 small shredded carrot
3 cups green cabbage – shredded
¼ cup minced onion
1 tablespoon vinegar
1/3 cup mayonnaise
2 teaspoons sugar
½ teaspoon each:
- Celery seed
- Salt

Instructions
1. Prepare the onion, carrots, and cabbage into a bowl.
2. Mix the dressing and pour over the slaw.

Yields: Six servings
Cal: 71.7 | P: 0.8 g | C: 7.9 g | F: 4.5 g

Cucumber and Onion Salad with Vinegar

Ingredients
Pinch of salt and pepper
1 red onion
3-5 cucumbers (peeled)
½ cup each:
- White vinegar
- Water
1/3 cup sugar

Instructions
1. Slice the cucumbers and onions very thin and add to a salad dish.

2. Combine the water, vinegar, salt, pepper, and sugar and pour over the veggies.
3. Add a cover and marinate for a minimum of one hour.

Yields: Six servings
Cal: 67.5 | P: 1.3 g | C: 16.9 g | F: 0.2 g

Eggplant Pesto Mini Pizza

Ingredients
1 each chopped:
- Bell pepper
- Tomato
- Eggplant

1 medium sliced red onion
1/8 teaspoon salt
3 cloves of garlic
Pinch of oregano
¼ cup each:
- Extra-virgin olive oil
- Pesto sauce
- Hummus

Vegan Parmesan cheese
Sandwich thins – Arnold Orowheat used
Optional: Pepper flakes

Instructions
1. Set the oven to 400°F.
2. Chop the vegetables and combine the oil, pepper, salt, oregano, and pepper flakes if desired. Arrange on a baking tin and toast for approximately 30 to 45 minutes or until they are done the way you like them.
3. Toast the buns and spread the hummus on them, add the veggies, and a bit of pesto sauce. Sprinkle with the vegan cheese and enjoy.

Yields: Four servings
Cal: 405| P: 11.4 g | C: 40.6 g | F: 24.5 g

Lentil Vegetarian Loaf

Ingredients
1 ½ cups rinsed – dried lentils
2 yellow onions
3 cups cooked brown rice
2 tablespoons canola/olive oil
½ cup ketchup
1 can tomato paste (6 ounces)
1 teaspoon each of:
   ▪ Marjoram
   ▪ Garlic powder
   ▪ Sage
½ cup - quartered cherry tomatoes
¾ cup tomato/pasta sauce
To Taste:
   ▪ Salt
   ▪ More ketchup

Instructions
   1. Preheat the oven to 350°F.
   2. Rinse and cook the lentils in 3 to 4 cups of water for approximately 30 minutes.
   3. Drain and slightly mash the lentils.
   4. Peel and chop the onions. Cook in the oil until golden.
   5. Combine the onions, lentils, tomato paste, rice, tomatoes, sauce and spices into a large pot. Mix well.
   6. Press the mixture into a well-greased baking dish with ½ cup of ketchup over the top.
   7. Bake for one hour.

Yields: Ten servings

Cal: 254.2 | P: 10.9 g | C: 44.9 g | F: 4.4 g

Spicy Sweet Potato Fries

Ingredients
1 ½ tablespoons olive oil
2 medium sweet potatoes
¼ teaspoon salt
1 teaspoon ground cumin
½ teaspoon each:
- Onion powder
- Chili powder

Instructions
1. Program the oven setting to 450°F.
2. Wash and cut the potatoes lengthwise into fry strips. Combine all ingredients together in a dish and shake
3. Arrange them on a baking sheet on some parchment paper or foil.
4. Bake and turn every 5 to 6 minutes - for a total of 20 minutes cooking time.

Yields: Four servings
Cal: 116.9 | P: 1.2 g | C: 16.4g | F: 5.4 g

Spinach Lasagna

Ingredients
1 large egg
2 cups cottage cheese (1% milkfat)
2 cups part-skim mozzarella cheese
10 ounces baby spinach
1 jar spaghetti/marinara tomato sauce
1 cup water
9 lasagna noodles

1/8 teaspoon black pepper

Instructions
1. Program the oven temperature to 350°F.
2. Combine the thawed, drained spinach, one cup of mozzarella, cottage cheese, egg, and the seasonings in a large mixing bowl.
3. Spray a 9x13x2-inch casserole dish with some cooking spray.
4. Layer ½ cup of the sauce, 3 noodles, and ½ of the cheese mixture. Repeat, and top with the noodles one cup of mozzarella. Pour water around the edges and toothpicks on top to place a piece of foil over the noodles.
5. Bake covered for one hour to 1 ½ hours. Let it rest 15 minutes.

Yields: Eight servings
Cal: 316.8 | P: 26.4 g | C: 24.3 g | F: 12.6 g

Squash and Apple Bake

Ingredients
2 medium apples
1 medium butternut squash
1 tablespoon each:
- Splenda
- All-purpose flour

½ teaspoon salt
¼ cup melted butter
2 teaspoons ground cinnamon

Instructions
1. Program the oven temperature to 350°F.
2. Peel and core the apples and cut them into thin wedges. Peel and cut the squash into ¾-inch cubes.

3. Combine the squash and apples together in a baking dish.
4. Add the remainder of ingredients together and add to the top of the mixed apples and squash.
5. Bake for 50 to 60 minutes in a covered dish. For the last ten minutes, you can remove the top if you prefer the topping crispier.

Yields: Six servings
Cal: 133 | P: 1 g | C: 17 g | F: 8 g

Vegetarian Chili

Ingredients
1 can (15 ounces) each:
- Dark red kidney beans
- Pinto beans
- Light red kidney beans
- Black beans

2 cans (28 ounces) crushed tomatoes
1 can (28 ounces) diced tomatoes
3 cups celery
1 small diced each of bell peppers:
- Yellow
- Red

1 medium red onion
4 tablespoons chili powder
3 tablespoons garlic powder
2 tablespoons ground cumin

Instructions
1. Drain and rinse all of the beans. Dice the veggies.
2. Lightly spray a large pan on the stovetop using medium heat and cook the veggies about six to seven minutes or until they are softened.

3. Combine the spices, beans, and tomatoes in a slow cooker or a Dutch oven.

Yields: Eight servings
Cal: 279.8 | P: 14.7 g | C: 58.4 g | F: 2.2 g

Vegetarian Frittata

Ingredients
6 ounces button mushrooms
1 pound asparagus
1 shallot
1 garlic clove
1 tablespoon olive oil
1 small zucchini
6 large eggs
1/3 cup 1% milk
¼ teaspoon of freshly ground black pepper
1 teaspoon salt
1 tablespoon chopped chives
Dash of nutmeg
2 medium/1 large tomato
¼ cup freshly grated parmesan cheese

Instructions
1. Set the oven temperature to 350°F.
2. *Prepare the Asparagus*: Wash and trim cutting it into one-inch pieces. Blanche the cut asparagus for one to two minutes. Shock it by adding it to ice water. Drain and set to the side.
3. Wash and slice the mushrooms. Saute them in the oil for ten minutes using medium heat. Mince the shallots and garlic and add – cooking two more minutes. Transfer the mushrooms to a plate and set aside.
4. Slice the zucchini lengthwise and into half-moon shapes.

5. Whisk the eggs, milk, chives, pepper, salt, and nutmeg in a large mixing dish. Add the mushroom mixture, asparagus, and zucchini.
6. Spray a two-quart baking dish with cooking spray and add the egg/veggie mixture.
7. Arrange the thinly sliced tomatoes on top and sprinkle with the parmesan cheese.
8. Bake 30-35 minutes. You can place the frittata under the broiler for two to three minutes to brown the top.
9. Cool and serve at room temperature or straight from the fridge.

Yields: Six servings
Cal: 146.2 | P: 10.6 g | C: 7.4 g | F: 8.8 g

Veggies with Grilled Pineapple

Ingredients
1 cup of each:
- Diced potatoes
- Bell peppers
- Raw mushrooms

1 cup cherry tomatoes
1 medium chopped onion
1 can of pineapple chunks – natural juices
2 teaspoons each:
- Dill weed
- Chopped garlic

1 teaspoon celery seed/salt
3 tablespoons olive oil
1 ½ teaspoons each: *Optional*:
- Onion powder
- Cayenne pepper
- Garlic powder

Pepper and salt to taste

Instructions

1. *Chop the veggies*
2. *Option 1*: Add the veggies on a piece of oil sprayed foil. Arrange the package on the grill using medium heat for 20-25 minutes (turning every five minutes).
3. *Option 2*: Place the veggies on wooden skewers that have been soaked in water. Cook on a med-high grill, turning every five minutes or so.
4. *Oven:* Bake at 400°F, checking every 10 minutes.

Yields: Six servings
Cal: 136.5 | P: 2.3 g | C: 17.0 g | F: 7.2 g

Fruit Salads

Caprese Salad

Ingredients
6 ounces strawberries
1 ripe avocado
1 (7 ounces) sliced mozzarella ball
Small handful salad leaves
2-3 tablespoons balsamic dressing – your choice
Pepper and salt

Instructions
1. Toss in the salad leaves, avocado, strawberries, and cheese into a serving dish.
2. Add the tasty dressing and sprinkle with the pepper and salt. Gently toss and enjoy.

Yields: Two servings
Cal: 375| P: 23.8g | C: 13 g| F: 24.6 g

California Roll in a Bowl

Ingredients
1 head chopped lettuce
1 cup cooked brown rice
1 English cucumber – seedless – thinly sliced
1 (8 ounces) package cooked shrimp/crabmeat – chopped
1 grated carrot
1 ripe diced avocado
3 tablespoons pickled ginger

Ingredients for the Dressing
1 tablespoon light soy sauce
½ teaspoon wasabi powder – to taste
3 tablespoons rice wine vinegar

Garnishes:
1 large sheet seaweed/nori (toasted and in small bits)
1 tablespoon sesame seeds

Instructions
1. Combine each of the fixings for the dressing in a mixing dish and whisk well.
2. Divide it into four sections and enjoy.

Note: You can locate the ginger in the Asian section of the supermarket.

Yields: Four servings
Cal: 199.1 | P: 6.5 g | C: 27.3 g | F: 8.3 g

Caramel Apple Salad

Ingredients
1 tub (8 ounces) Cool Whip Free

1 box Instant Butter Scotch Pudding mix (sugar-free)
1 can (14 ounces) pineapple tidbits with the juice
4 large each:

- Fuji apples/Red Delicious
- Granny Smith apples

Instructions
1. Mix the pineapple with its juice and the pudding mix in a large mixing container.
2. Dice the apples into small portions and fold in the Cool Whip.
3. Mix well, and chill in the refrigerator until ready to eat.

Yields: 16 servings
Cal: 90.7 | P: 0.2 g | C: 20.1 g | F: 0.4 g

Grape Salad

Ingredients
2-4 pounds of grapes (green, red, or both)
1 package of fat-free– 8 ounces each:

- Sour cream
- Softened cream cheese

½ cup each:

- Splenda/your choice
- Walnuts/Pecans

¼ cup brown sugar
4 tablespoons vanilla extract

Instructions
1. Wash and drain the grapes.
2. Combine the sour cream, cream cheese, vanilla, and sugar—blending well for about three to four minutes on high with a mixer.
3. Toss in the grapes and toss until covered.

4. Pour into a 9x13 cake pan. Sprinkle lightly with the brown sugar. Add the nuts.
5. Chill about one hour before serving.

Yields: 16 servings
Cal: 133.7 | P: 2.7 g | C: 18.4 g | F: 5.9 g

Israeli Salad

Ingredients

1 medium peeled cucumber
3 medium tomatoes
1 yellow/green bell pepper
2 tbsp. lemon juice
3 tbsp. extra-virgin olive oil
1 tsp. of salt and fresh ground pepper

Instructions

1. Chop all of the veggies into small bits.
2. Combine the rest of the ingredients and enjoy.

Yields: Eight servings
Cal: 65.2 | P: 0.8 g | C: 4.4 g | F: 5.6g

Sunshine Fruit Salad

Ingredients

2 cans (15 ounces each) mandarin oranges in light syrup
3 cans (20 ounces each) pineapple chunks in 100% juice
2 large bananas
3 medium kiwi fruits – bite-sized

Instructions

1. Drain the oranges and pineapple. Reserve the pineapple juice.

2. Combine all of the fruit (omit the bananas).
3. Submerge the fruit with the juice and chill for a minimum of one hour.
4. Slice and stir in the bananas before serving.

Yields: 10 servings
Cal: 135.2 | P: 1.5 g | C: 34.6 g | F: 0.4 g

Chapter 7: Snacks and Desserts

Black Bean Brownies

Ingredients
4 large eggs
1 can (15 ounces) black beans
3 tablespoons cocoa powder
½ cup granulated Splenda
1 tablespoon instant coffee*
2 tablespoons olive/canola oil
1 teaspoon each:
- Baking powder
- Vanilla

Instructions
1. Set the oven temperature to 350°F. Spray an 8x8 pan with some non-stick cooking spray.
2. *Dissolve the coffee in one tablespoon of hot water and mix with the rest of the ingredients. Drain and rinse the black beans, adding them last.
3. Bake 30 minutes, and perform the toothpick test for doneness.
4. Let cool before slicing into 2x2-inch brownies.

Yields: 16 servings
Cal: 79.2 | P: 4.1 g | C: 8.9 g | F: 3.4 g

Blueberry Muffin

Ingredients
1 cup of each:
- Flour
- Old-fashioned oats
1 tsp. each:

- Cinnamon
- Baking soda

½ tsp. of salt

½ cup each:
- Unsweetened applesauce
- Water
- Sugar

2 egg whites

1 cup frozen blueberries

Instructions
1. Prepare 12 muffin tins and program the oven to 350°F.
2. Combine the salt, soda, cinnamon, oats, and flour.
3. Add the egg whites, sugar, water, and applesauce.
4. Blend in the blueberries
5. Bake 20 to 25 minutes until lightly browned.

Yields: 12 servings

Cal: 102.8 | P: 3.1 g | C: 21.9 g | F: 0.9 g

Coconut Meringue Cookies

Ingredients

2 egg whites

1 ½ cups sweetened shredded coconut

Dash of salt

2/3 cup granulated sugar

¼ teaspoon vanilla extract

Instructions
1. Whip the eggs with a dash of salt to form stiff peaks. Stir in the sugar and fold in the coconut.
2. Drop by teaspoons onto a lightly greased cookie sheet.
3. Bake 18 to20 minutes at 325°F.

Yields: 20 servings
Cal: 50.6 | P: 0.5 g | C: 8.4 g | F: 1.8 g

Healthy Breakfast Cookie

Ingredients
2 large eggs
¼ cup butter
½ cup each:
- Honey
- Chopped - dried apricots
- Raisins

1 cup each:
- Grated carrots
- Chopped walnuts
- All-purpose flour
- Rolled oats

1 ½ cups Cheerios
1 teaspoon each:
- Cinnamon
- Nutmeg

Instructions
1. Mix the butter, honey, and egg in a mixing bowl. Combine the mixture with the apricots, walnuts, and raisins.
2. In a separate container, mix the cinnamon, nutmeg, flour, and oats.
3. Combine all components and mix well. Fold in the Cheerios.
4. Drop the dough onto a baking sheet about one inch apart.
5. Bake 15 minutes or until the cookie is firm.

Yields: 30 servings
Cal: 111.1 | P: 2.1 g | C: 16.2 g | F: 5.0 g

Mini Cheesecakes

Ingredients
3 ounces cream cheese
12 ounces fat-free cream cheese
12 low-fat vanilla wafers
½ teaspoon vanilla
½ cup sugar
2 eggs
Cherry pie filling

Instructions
1. Set the oven temperature to 350°F.
2. Let the cream cheese sit out at room temperature.
3. Line 12 muffin tins with foil cake liners and add a wafer to each one.
4. Combine the regular and fat-free cheese until smooth. Blend in the sugar, vanilla, and eggs – beating until smooth.
5. Pour the batter into the tins and bake for 20 minutes.
6. Refrigerate for a minimum of two hours – preferably overnight.
7. Add the cherry filling to each one and serve.

Yields: 12 mini cakes
Cal: 119.3 | P: 6 g | C: 14.5 g | F: 4.4 g

Pumpkin Muffins

Ingredients
1 can/1 pound pumpkin
½ cup flaxseed meal
1 box spice cake mix

Instructions

1. Program the oven to 350°F.
2. Line a muffin tin with paper liners or cooking spray.
3. Combine all of the ingredients and bake 25 minutes.
4. Check for doneness with a toothpick in the center. If it comes out clean – it's done.
5. Enjoy when you just don't have time for the 'from scratch' recipe.

Yields: 18 servings
Cal: 340 | P: 6 g | C: 53.0g | F: 12.5 g

Cold Goodies

Mixed Berry Smoothie

Ingredients
1 cup of each:
- Skim milk
- Fat-free yogurt

¾ cup frozen assorted berries/your choice
Optional: ¼ cup sugar

Instructions
1. Empty the yogurt and milk into a blender along with the berries.
2. Add some protein powder if you choose and enjoy.

Yields: Two servings
Cal: 257.8| P: 11.1 g |C: 47.4 g | F: 2.8 g

Pumpkin Mousse

Ingredients
1 can (15 ounces) pumpkin
1 package (4 ounces) fat-free vanilla pudding
½ cup skim milk

2 cups sugar-free whipped topping
1 teaspoon cinnamon
Possible Additions
- Nutmeg
- Ginger
- Allspice
- Clove
- Splenda

Instructions
1. Combine all of the ingredients together and whip until smooth.

Yields: Four servings
Cal: 149 | P: 2 g | C: 28 g | F: 3.4 g

Yogurt Breakfast Popsicles

Ingredients
1 cup of each:
- Chopped fruits/mixed berries
- Plain non-fat Greek yogurt

½ cup each:
- Instant/regular oats
- Skim/1% milk

Also Needed: Popsicle molds

Instructions
1. Combine the yogurt and milk and pour into two molds.
2. Add a few berries to each one along with half of the oatmeal.
3. Add an ice cream stick to each mold and freeze for a minimum of four hours.

Yields: Six servings
Cal: 75 | P: 5 g | C: 11 g | F: 0.6 g

Conclusion

Thank for making it through to the end of *Bariatric Cookbook: Delicious Recipes to Recover Yourself After Bariatric Weight Loss Surgery*. Let's hope it was informative and provided you with all of the tools you need to achieve your goals whatever they may be.

The next step is to set up your dietary meal plans and get the cabinets stocked with the nutritious foods you will need to get your life on the right track and make healthier choices for you and your family.

Losing weight and making a bright future is not always eating dull and tasteless meals as you will soon discover. Finally, if you found this book useful in any way, a review on Amazon is always appreciated!

Index

Chapter 1: Poultry and Turkey

Chapter 2: Seafood

Salmon

Shrimp

- Veggies with Grilled Pineapple

Fruit Salads
- Caprese Salad
- California Roll in a Bowl
- Caramel Apple Salad
- Grape Salad
- Israeli Salad
- Sunshine Fruit Salad

Chapter 7: Snacks and Desserts

- Black Bean Brownies
- Blueberry Muffin
- Coconut Meringue Cookies
- Healthy Breakfast Cookie
- Mini Cheesecakes
- Pumpkin Muffins

Cold Goodies
- Mixed Berry Smoothie
- Pumpkin Mousse
- Yogurt Breakfast Popsicles

www.ingramcontent.com/pod-product-compliance
Lightning Source LLC
Chambersburg PA
CBHW071221220526
45468CB00002B/696